Cancer Early Symptoms: How to Detect the Warning Signs

Book Description

It is estimated that one in four people will be diagnosed with some form of cancer in their lifetime. Cancer is a disease which is likely to touch all of our lives, either personally or by affecting a loved one or family member. The good news is that treatment and detection methods are improving every day, and there is now a greater than fifty per cent survival rate for those diagnosed with cancer. The figures for some types, including some of the most common forms, are even higher.

Early detection is one of the most important keys to successful treatment. In this book we will look at some of the early warning signs of the commonest forms of cancer, including:

- Breast cancer
- Lung cancer
- Prostate cancer
- Bowel cancer
- Malignant melanoma
- Cervical cancer

Along with some simple signs to be aware of, we will also discuss some preventative steps you can take, as well as what to do if you think you or someone close to you may be showing some of the warning signs. Cancer is a serious disease, but with information, prompt treatment and good medical care, you can give yourself or someone close to you the best chance of survival.

Introduction

If you do find any of the signs of any type of cancer, the first thing to remember is that there is no need to panic. The majority of cancer signs turn out to be benign and the best thing you can do is to get prompt medical attention to put your mind at rest. You will not be 'wasting the doctor's time' or making a fuss. The majority of cancers can be tested for quickly and simply, and your doctor will be able be advise you on the best course of action.

Similarly, if you think you spot any worrying symptoms in someone close to you, the best thing to do is to let them know that you are concerned. There is no need to frighten them, but do ask them, as a personal favor to you, to get it checked out. If it is your partner, then feel free to nag them until they go. It is well known that people in long-term relationships live longer than single people, and a great deal of this is due to having someone else keeping an eye on you and noticing any changes to your body. Especially with things like changes to moles or freckles, the symptom may be in a place that you yourself cannot easily see, or may have come on so slowly that you have not noticed the change.

If you yourself spot something on another person that you think they ought to have checked, then do so sensitively, and offer to come along with them to the doctor. Part of taking care of a partner, family member or friend is to act with their best interests at heart.

If you are diagnosed with cancer, then remember that your chances of survival are good and that everyone around you wants to help. Your medical professionals will give you the best possible care, and you can accept the love and support of the people close to you. Don't let your fear of cancer stop you from seeking prompt medical attention — it gives you the best chance of shortening the treatment you will receive.

Chapter 1 – Breast Cancer

Breast cancer is the most common form of cancer in women. However, the survival rate for breast cancer in the UK is currently at over eighty five per cent. Men are also at risk and, although the rates are much lower, it is something that everyone, male or female, should be aware of.

Most people think of the classic symptom of breast cancer to be a lump in the breast tissue. If you do discover a lump or area of thickened tissue in your breast, the best thing to do is to have it checked out by your doctor. Bear in mind that eighty per cent of lumps are entirely benign, so there is no need to panic, but you should get it checked as soon as possible.

Other signs include:

- A change to one or both nipples, including darkening, inversion (where the nipple starts to point inwards rather than out) or any discharge from the nipple when gently squeezed.

- Any appearance of puckering to the skin of the breast, or a rash around your nipple, even if there is no itching or discomfort.

- A lump in one or both armpits

- A change in size of one or other breast

The best way to be aware of any changes to your breasts is to examine them regularly. Put one arm above your head and use the other hand to gently massage your breast tissue, starting from the armpit and moving to the bottom of the breast. Gently squeeze each nipple to check for any discharge.

Women should get to know their breasts, especially any changes to size and shape that may occur throughout the menstrual cycle. Get into the habit of checking your breasts every day, or at the same point in your menstrual cycle.

Risk factors for breasts cancer are quite widespread, although the following may increase your chances:

- Alcohol. If you think your alcohol consumption is above health guidelines and you feel it would be difficult to cut down, you can ask your GP for help. Many areas run programs to help you reduce (rather than just eliminate) your alcohol consumption and remember that you deserve help and support in improving your overall health.

- Long-term use of estrogen-based contraceptives or HRT. The risks of these should be weighed up with the advantages of taking them — the pill is an excellent long-term contraceptive and there are many downsides associated with an unplanned pregnancy. The use of the pill should be a reason to check your breasts, rather than a reason to come off it in order to reduce the risk of breast cancer.

- Being overweight
- High exposure to gamma rays and x rays. Most people have a few x rays in their lifetime — again, this is a reason to be vigilant, not a reason to avoid x rays.
- There is some evidence that long-term shiftwork which requires you to constantly readjust your body clock may put you at higher risk of developing breast cancer as well as a few other forms.
- Age. Women who are past the age of menopause are more than twice as likely to develop breast cancer as women who are still menstruating.
- There is also evidence that the risk for breast cancer can be hereditary. If you have a close family member, of a history of breast cancer in your family, you should be extra vigilant. There is also a test for the so-called 'breast cancer gene' which some people elect to be screened for, however, the majority of breast cancer cases are not linked to genetic factors.

Some factors, such as having breastfed or the number of live births a woman goes through, would seem to reduce the chances of breast cancer. Again, these should not be seen as protecting you from ever getting breast cancer, and everyone should still be aware of any changes to the breast tissue.

If you think you have any of the signs of breast cancer you should visit your GP. He or she will probably refer you to a specialist breast clinic, where they will use one or more of the following tests to examine your breasts:

- A mammogram: This is a low-dose x-ray of the breast and is usually only carried out on women over thirty five. The breast needs to be slightly flattened for this to be effective, and women with denser breasts may find this uncomfortable, even painful.
- A breast ultrasound: this is a painless test which uses sound waves to build up a picture of the tissues inside the breast and lymph nodes in the armpit.
- A biopsy. This is where a small piece of tissue is removed from the inside of the breast, which can then be analyzed in a lab. There are several methods of obtaining a tissue sample (depending on the location and size of the lump), many of which are performed under local anesthetic.

Some of the results of these tests will be supplied to you on the day and some may take as much as a few weeks to come back. If you do have to wait for your results, discuss any anxieties you feel with your health workers and ask the people close to you for their support.

Breast cancer survival rates are high, and the earlier it is detected, the less likely it is that you will require a full mastectomy. Partial removal of breasts tissue followed by radiotherapy has been shown to as effective as a full mastectomy in treating early-stage breast cancer.

Chapter 2 – Prostate Cancer

Prostate cancer is the most common cancer in men. The prostate is a gland in the pelvis which is located between the bladder and penis, (found only in men) and its function is to produce seminal fluid. Although this type of cancer is common, it takes time to develop and it is usually only diagnosed when it becomes large enough to put pressure on the urethra.

The symptoms of prostate cancer include:

- needing to urinate more often. Many men start to notice that they are waking up more frequently during the night to use the toilet
- needing to rush to the toilet due to a sudden, strong urge
- difficulty in starting to urinate
- straining or taking a long time while urinating
- weak flow of urine
- even after you have been to the toilet, still feeling that your bladder has not emptied fully

If you experience any of these symptoms it is more likely to be caused by something else rather than cancer. Many men's prostates naturally enlarge as they age and this is more likely to be benign than malignant. However, any changes to your toilet habits or anything which causes you discomfort or inconvenience should be checked out by your doctor.

There are a number of factors that are thought to increase your risk of developing prostate cancer, which include:

- Age. The majority of men diagnosed with prostate cancer are over fifty.
- Obesity. Men with a higher percentage of body fat are at greater risk.
- Family history. Having a close male relative who is diagnosed with prostate cancer would seem to elevate your risk. There is some evidence that having a close female relative who develops breast cancer can also increase your risk.
- Ethic group. Men from African and Afro-Caribbean backgrounds are more at risk from prostate cancer. Men from Asian and South and Central American backgrounds would seem to be at lower risk.
- There is some evidence that a higher consumption of calcium-rich foods can increase your risk of developing prostate cancer.

Men over the age of fifty are routinely offered a prostate exam by their GP. This is a digital rectal exam, in which the doctor inserts their gloved and lubricated finger into the rectum to check the surface of the prostate through the rectal wall. Although it can be a little uncomfortable, it is brief and painless. The doctor will be checking for changes to the smoothness of the prostate — any lumps or bumps may indicate changes which should be monitored. A benign enlargement of the prostate will result in it having a smooth surface.

If you have any of the symptoms of prostate cancer, the doctor may also need to perform a few tests to rule out other factors:

- A urine sample will be taken to rule out bladder infections, which are the most common cause of frequent urination. This is easily treated with a course of antibiotics.
- A blood sample to check levels of prostate-specific antigen — this can act as a 'marker' for the presence of certain types of cancer
- An ultrasound-guided biopsy. This is where an ultrasound probe is used to guide a small needle into the prostate to take a sample of tissue. This can sometimes be painful, so is usually performed under local anaesthetic.

Even if you are diagnosed with prostate cancer, there may be no need for immediate treatment. Prostate cancer is very slow growing, and the most likely course of action your doctor will suggest is that the prostate should be regularly monitored. If treatment is needed, there are a number of options your health care workers can discuss to see what would be the most appropriate for you.

Chapter 3 – Lung Cancer

Lung cancer is one of the most common forms of cancer, and around 90 per cent of cases are attributable to environmental factors — most commonly smoking. It is also a relatively dangerous form of cancer, with fewer than one in ten people living for more than five years after diagnosis.

Lung cancer often causes no symptoms in the early stages, but later effects include:

- a persistent cough (longer than three weeks) or an existing cough that gets worse
- coughing up blood
- persistent breathlessness, especially when exercising or climbing stairs
- unexplained tiredness and weight loss
- an ache or pain in the chest when breathing or coughing
- A less common symptom can be to notice 'clubbing' to the ends of your fingers. This is when the fingers become more curved and the fingertips become enlarged.

Although the majority of cases are diagnosed in smokers, you should not ignore any of these symptoms even if you have never smoked. Other risk factors include:

- Passive smoking. There is some evidence to suggest that living with a partner who smokes increases your risk of lung cancer
- Exposure to Radon gas. This is a naturally occurring radioactive gas that is present in some areas of the country, and can build up in certain buildings. This is thought to be responsible for up to three per cent of lung cancer cases but may be much higher, since the risks of smoking 'drown out' the other factors and make them harder to ascertain
- Environmental exposure to other pollutants, including asbestos, arsenic, coal fumes and silica

If you have any of these symptoms, you should visit your doctor. He or she will ask you a few questions about your general health and may check your lung flow (using a device called a spirometer) and take a blood test to rule out a chest infection. Other diagnostic tests include:

- A chest x-ray. This will check for any unusual masses in your lungs, which can then be investigated further.
- A CT scan. This can investigate your chest in more detail and requires a harmless dye to be added to your lungs to make them show up more clearly on the scan.

If the scans show any cause for concern, you may be given a biopsy to remove a small piece of tissue from your lung. Although this involves a tube being fed down your nose into your lung and can be a little uncomfortable, you will be given a mild sedative and local anaesthetic so it should not be painful, and should not take more than a few minutes.

Chapter 4 – Bowel Cancer

Bowel cancer is another common cancer, with around one in twenty people in the UK likely to develop the disease in their lifetime. Bowel cancer is a general term for cancers which develop in the large bowel. Depending on the location, it is sometimes called rectal or colon cancer. More than half of people diagnosed with bowel cancer will live at least ten years after diagnosis.

To reduce your risk of bowel cancer, you are advised to make sure your diet includes plenty of roughage, and try to limit your consumption of red meat, especially cured or processed meat. Try to maintain a healthy weight and keep alcohol consumption within health guidelines. In addition, in the UK everyone aged between sixty and seventy four will be offered free bowel cancer screening by their GP. Usually this consists of a non-invasive stool sample, which can be collected at home and posted off in a sealed envelope.

The three main symptoms of bowel cancer are:

- Blood in your stools
- Abdominal pain
- Persistent changes to bowel habit, including loose stools.

These are extremely common symptoms and can be caused by a range of factors. For example, blood in your stool is most likely to be caused by hemorrhoids and loose stools by something you have eaten, changes to your diet or a stomach virus.

One of the biggest risk factors is age, with the majority of diagnoses being made in people over sixty, so more attention should be paid to these symptoms in older people. Another, less common, symptom is abdominal pain, discomfort or bloating after eating. This may lead to a reduction in food consumed and subsequent weight loss

Very rarely, bowel cancer can cause an obstruction in your bowel. This is when the bowel becomes partially or completely blocked and feces can no longer exit the body. The symptoms of this are severe abdominal pain, being unable to pass stools, vomiting and swelling of the abdomen. If you suspect you have a bowel obstruction you should regard this as a serious medical emergency and seek help immediately.

If you are concerned that you may have bowel cancer, your doctor will initially perform an examination of your abdomen and rectal area and take a blood test to check for anemia — this may be caused by bleeding higher up the bowel of which you are unaware. You may also be referred to a hospital or clinic for a rectal sigmoidoscopy. This is a tiny camera on a flexible tube which is inserted into your rectum and used to check your bowel. A biopsy may also be taken.

If you are given the all clear but symptoms persist, you can ask to be checked again. Bowel health is important and should not be a source of embarrassment or reluctance to seek treatment.

Chapter 5 – Malignant Melanoma

This is more commonly referred to as skin cancer, and is much rarer than the other forms of cancer we have discussed. However, incidents are on the rise and it is now the fifth most common cancer in the UK. Skin cancer is usually simple to treat, but can spread to other organs of the body, so should be taken seriously.

The most common sign of melanoma is a new mole appearing or changes to an existing mole. People with fairer skins, red or blonde hair, blue eyes, lots of existing moles, a history of sunburn or a close relative with skin cancer are more at risk. There are also rarer risk factors, including:

- Damage to skin caused by radiotherapy treatment
- A condition which causes suppression of the immune system such as HIV or certain types of medication (such as those prescribed following an organ transplant)
- Expose to certain chemicals such as arsenic or creosote

Everyone should try to avoid sunburn. If you are light skinned then you should wear sunscreen, cover up with loose clothing and avoid sunbathing, especially at midday or in strong sunlight. There is also evidence linking the use of sunbeds to an increased risk of skin cancer. If you have been sunburnt even once in your life, you are more than twice as likely to develop melanoma than someone who has never been burned.

You should keep an eye on your moles and familiarize yourself with their shape and color. If you have one or more of the risk factors, it is a good idea to ask a friend or partner to periodically check areas of your body such as your back, which may have moles you cannot monitor. If you spot a mole on someone else which you feel is concerning, then mention it to them. There is no need to panic them, but let them know they ought to keep an eye on it. If you have a lot of moles or ones of particular concern, you may like to photograph them so you can make an accurate comparison.

Changes to moles to look out for are sometimes referred to as the ABCDE checklist:

- **A**symmetrical – melanomas can have two very different halves and are an irregular shape rather than round.
- **B**order – melanomas have a notched or ragged border.
- **C**olours – melanomas will be a mix of two or more colours.
- **D**iameter – melanomas are larger than 6mm (1/4 inch) in diameter.

- **Enlargement or elevation** – a mole that changes size over time is more likely to be a melanoma.

If you are concerned about changes to a mole, your GP can examine you and refer you to a specialist. The most common treatment will be to remove the mole under local anaesthetic and send it for laboratory testing to check if it was cancerous. If this test comes back positive, you may require further treatment.

If you are given the all-clear, you should still continue to check your moles and return to your doctor if you notice further changes.

Chapter 6 – Cervical Cancer

Cervical cancer is a rare and slow-growing form of cancer that develops at the cervix, which is at the neck of the uterus. It is advised that all women over the age of twenty-five should be routinely tested for abnormal cervical cells — this is commonly called a smear test.

Cervical cancer is unlikely to produce any symptoms in the early stages and so is mostly diagnosed during routine testing. The main symptom is irregular bleeding between periods or after penetrative sex , along with abdominal pain. If you experience either of these symptoms then you should visit your GP, but there is no need to panic — these symptoms are more likely to be caused by something else such as an infection.

The cervical smear is a procedure in which a speculum is inserted into the vagina and a small swab is used to gather cells from the cervix which can then be sent away for testing. It can be uncomfortable but should be over very quickly.

If these cells show any abnormalities which may be at risk of developing into cancer, then you may be referred for a colposcopy. This is a more detailed examination of the cervix, again performed using a speculum. A solution may be applied to the cervix to make precancerous cells more visible, and a biopsy may be taken of any areas of concern. This is painful but brief. You may also experience soreness, bleeding and abdominal pain afterwards, but this can be treated with over-the-counter painkillers and a sanitary towel. It is not advised that you insert anything into the vagina for three days after the procedure.

Cervical cancer is most often caused by the Human Papiloma Virus. This is a very common virus, present in a great number of the population. There are over a hundred different strains, most of which are harmless but a few are linked to the development of diseases such as genital warts, herpes and cancer. It is most often spread via sex, and although condoms offer some protection, they are not 100 per cent effective. Fortunately a vaccine has been developed against the most dangerous strains, and is now routinely offered to girls between the ages of twelve and thirteen. This vaccine is most effective if administered before someone becomes sexually active and is also safe for boys to take. However, most people with the virus will shed it within a few years of infection, and most do not go on to develop any cancerous symptoms.

Chapter 7 — Non Hodgkins' Lymphoma

This is a rarer form of cancer which affects the lymphatic system. Because of this, it can compromise your immune system and make you more vulnerable to infection.

The most common symptom of NHL is a painless swelling in the neck, armpit of groin. Some other, rarer symptoms include:

- night sweats
- unexplained weight loss
- a high temperature
- persistent tiredness or fatigue
- difficulty recovering from illness or minor infections
- persistent itching of the skin all over the body

No one really knows what causes NHL to develop, but some risk factors may include:

- having a medical condition that weakens your immune system, such as HIV, taking medication that suppresses your immune system (for example, following an organ transplant) or having an autoimmune condition such as lupus or coeliac disease.
- being previously exposed to the Epstein-Barr virus (a common virus that causes glandular fever)
- having a Helicobacter pylori infection (a common bacterial infection that usually infects the lining of the stomach and small intestine)
- having received chemotherapy or radiotherapy for an earlier cancer

The risk of diagnosis increases with age, with most people being diagnosed over the age of fifty five.

If you have a persistent raised gland, even if you don't have any of the other symptoms, you should get it checked out by your GP. There is no need to panic — there are many causes of raised lymph glands and most are entirely harmless.

The doctor will examine you, ask a few questions about your health and may refer you for a biopsy. A sample will be taken from you lymph node, most often under local anesthetic and sent to a laboratory for testing.

There are around thirty different forms of NHL, and (if the biopsy shows evidence of concern) further tests may be carried out to ascertain the exact nature and stage of the NHL.

Types of non-Hodgkin's lymphoma can be put broadly into two groups: low-grade or high-grade. Low-grade NHL is by far the most common sort and is very slow-growing and often does not require immediate medical treatment. High-grade is more aggressive but responds better to treatment. It is possible for low-grade NHL to become high-grade NHL over time.

Because NHL affects the lymphatic system, it can sometimes cause complications such as making your body more vulnerable to other diseases and infections. You should be aware of this and take extra hygiene precautions to reduce your contact with pathogens. Your GP may also prescribe a protective course of antibiotics if you are suspected of having NHL. Keep an eye on any potential illnesses or infections you feel you may be developing. It is important also to make sure that your vaccinations are kept up to date, although you should check with your doctor before receiving any 'live' vaccinations (that is, vaccinations which contained weakened forms of the disease) if you are being treated for NHL. However, your immune system should gradually recover following successful treatment of NHL.

Chapter 8 — Testicular Cancer

Testicular cancer is uncommon, but is unusual in that it is most likely to affect young men between the ages of fifteen and forty five. Because of this, it is vital that young men are aware of the symptoms, since they may not be on the lookout for them.

The classic symptom of testicular cancer is a lump in one testicle. Men should regularly examine their testicles and check for any changes, lumps or swellings in their scrotum. Along with changes to the testicles you may also experience:

- intermittent pain or aching in the testicles or scrotum
- a feeling of heaviness in the scrotum
- a sudden collection of fluid in your scrotum (this is called a hydrocele)
- a general feeling of being unwell or tired

Although this is not a common form of cancer, parents should make sure that young men are aware of the signs to look out for and get into the habit of regularly checking their testicles.

If you do find a lump in your testicles, it is important to see your GP. Don't panic — the vast majority of lumps will turn out to be harmless swellings or cysts, but in the rare occasion that a lump is a cause for concern, the earlier the treatment, the more successful it will be.

The doctor will examine your testicles and scrotum, and may shine a light against your scrotum to see if the lump is solid. If he or she feels that you would benefit from further testing, you may be referred for one or more of the following:

- An ultrasound test to get a better picture of the tissues in the scrotum
- A blood test to detect certain 'markers' in your blood which may indicate the presence of cancer
- A biopsy of the lump itself. This is likely to be performed under local anaesthetic.

If it turns out that you do have testicular cancer, early treatment gives the best chance of a full recovery, with no damage to your sexual function or your ability to father children in the future.

Conclusion

We hope you have found this guide helpful and informative. We can all be more cancer aware, and just knowing what the signs are and looking out for them in ourselves and others could save a life.

If you have any concerns, your first port of call should be your GP. He or she can answer any questions and set your mind at rest, as well as supplying more detailed information for you to take away. If you are concerned about a symptom in someone close to you, urge them to make an appointment and offer to go with them to provide support.

Most of the symptoms of cancer turn out to be something much less serious and can be easily treated or mitigated. But do not use this as an excuse to avoid finding out for sure — you will feel much better when your doctor has confirmed for you that your symptoms are harmless or easy to treat.

If it does turn out that you receive a positive cancer diagnosis, remember that the survival rates for all types of cancer are improving every day. Your medical team want to provide the best possible care for you, and your friends or family will be on your side as well. There is lots of help and support out there for you, and you will not have to do this alone.

www.ingramcontent.com/pod-product-compliance
Lightning Source LLC
Chambersburg PA
CBHW030042230526
45472CB00002B/637